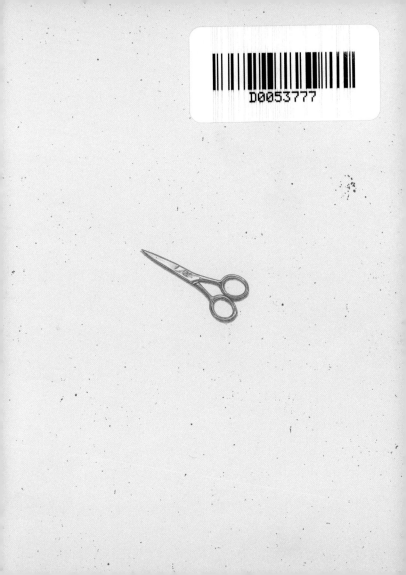

The
MOUSTACHE
GROWER'S
Guide

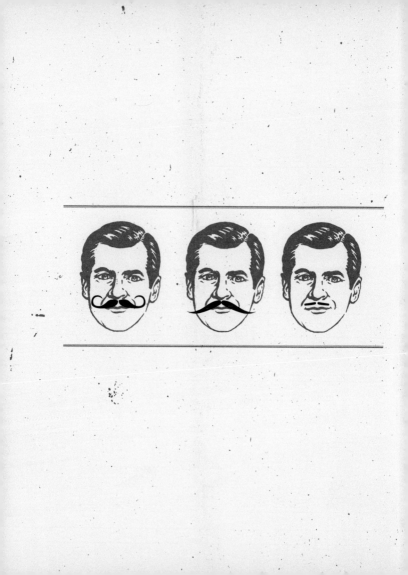

The MOUSTACHE GROWER'S Guide

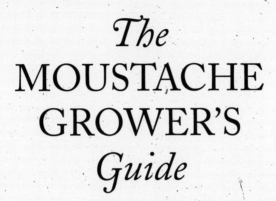

Lucien Edwards

CHRONICLE BOOKS
SAN FRANCISCO

Library of Congress Cataloging-in-Publication Data available.

ISBN: 978-0-8118-7880-7

Manufactured in China

Designed by Jacob T. Gardner

PHOTO CREDITS
Pages 34, 38, 62, 66, 96: Getty Images
Page 124: Jason Whalen
Page 128: Dave Mead
Page 132: Roger Holcombe
Page 136: Michael Elsden
Page 140: Matthew Rainwaters

Disclaimer: The author and publisher hereby disclaim any liability from any
injury that may result from the use, proper or improper, of the information
contained within this book. Exercise caution before using any facial hair-care tools,
appliances, products, or accessories.

10 9 8 7 6 5 4

Chronicle Books LLC
680 Second Street
San Francisco, CA 94107

www.chroniclebooks.com

"A man without a moustache is like a cup of tea without sugar."

— English proverb

Table of Contents

Moustache Combos

Championship Styles

INTRODUCTION

From prehistoric times to now, the moustache has evolved from a roughly hewn block of hair into a genuine work of art. An artist needs his tools, however, and over the years moustache connoisseurs have found help in a long parade of tools and accessories beginning with sharpened rocks and evolving to include waxes, scissors, razors, snoods (a moustache net used while sleeping), moustache cups (special drinking cups), and a host of others. Meanwhile, the popularity of the moustache in society has been a long journey full of ups and downs. Just when it seems that the 'stache has been resigned to the realm of fops and rogues (or, in modern times, porn stars), a cultural revolution will swing the pendulum back and usher in a new day for moustaches.

Regardless of its current standing in popular culture, the moustache will always be fashionable among those who can see through the fuzz and truly appreciate its subtle charms. This book is for them. Inside is information and instructions for shaving and maintaining a world of classic and modern moustache styles. Some take less time, some are more difficult, some require sticky waxes. All are a fun and creative way to put your whiskers to some use, so don't be bashful about trying any or every one of them.

As any dedicated moustache grower will tell you, however, it's not so important what kind of moustache you sport but how you wear it. Accordingly, much attention has been paid within these pages to inform the reader of appropriate attire for pairing with specific styles. These are only suggestions—readers are encouraged to dress their brush up in whatever outfits suit their fancy. Really the only thing one should absolutely not forget before leaving the house is self-confidence, which allows anyone to pull off even the most absurd costume.

No matter what style you wear or what outfit you put on, the most important thing is to have fun with your moustache. Twist, wax, snip, or trim—just imagine your whiskers as a clean palette on which to create your brilliant masterpiece.

HOW TO USE THIS BOOK

Each entry in this book provides a description of a unique style, instructions for sculpting and grooming, and suggestions for accompanying attire. Within each section, moustaches are ranked from easiest to most difficult. A note is also given for the approximate time it will take to grow each style. All instructions presuppose that readers have stopped shaving for the length of time indicated and have a full moustache and beard to work with. Those who are comfortable with this shaggy approach are encouraged to read the entry on the Lumberjack (p. 86) for suggestions on grooming and attire during the growing process. Others should simply continue shaving at regular intervals while following the instructions given. Depending on the rate of hair growth, the moustache will be complete in roughly the same amount of time.

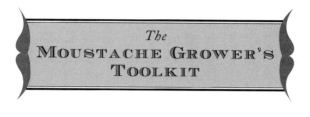

The MOUSTACHE GROWER'S TOOLKIT

Every artist needs the right tools in order to create a masterpiece. Use this list to familiarize yourself with the basics, then spend some time experimenting with different products to learn what works best for you.

RAZOR

The most important tool in your kit, razors come in a variety of styles. Use whichever feels most comfortable to you and always be sure to follow the manufacturer's instructions—this is your face we're talking about, after all.

Swivel Head Razor: The standard model for most men, these razors feature a disposable cartridge for the blades. The swivel head allows the blades to move with the contours of your face.

Fixed Head Razor: Think cheap, plastic, and disposable; the fixed head means limited mobility and the blades are generally only sharp enough for one shave.

Electric Razor: The choice of traveling businessmen and rushed morning commuters, electric razors allow for dry shaves on the go but don't offer as close a shave as a traditional wet-shave razor.

While you won't find the following razors in the aisles of a drugstore, you can still spot them on the cheeks of some professionals and shaving aficionados:

Safety Razor: Seldom used today, these old-school razors feature replaceable blades. Despite the safety razor's name, modern razors are actually much safer.

Straight Razor: With their single, sharp blades, these razors provide ultra–close shaves. Seek advice from an experienced professional before taking this model for a test–drive.

ELECTRIC TRIMMER

Featuring two comb-shaped blades that cut with to-the-millimeter accuracy, electric trimmers are indispensable for tricky or precision styles. Choose one with the maximum number of attachments (combs that attach to the trimmer and elevate the blades above the face), which allow you to trim large or small areas of hair to whatever height you choose.

MOUSTACHE SCISSORS

These small, sharp scissors are perfect for cleaning up rough edges and manual detailing.

MOUSTACHE COMB

This classic accessory features a small row of closely spaced teeth and is ideal for straightening out any tangled or unruly moustache hairs.

SHAVING BRUSH

While shaving brushes, which are used to apply traditional shaving cream, are less ubiquitous than they once were, serious shavers still swear by them. Aside from delivering a frothy, even lather onto your face, these brushes have the added benefit of massaging the skin, thereby relaxing the face and providing a superior shave. Choose those made of badger hair for a sublime experience.

CREAMS, SOAPS, FOAMS, AND GELS

Foams and gels often contain irritating chemicals. Traditional shaving creams and soaps, though not as easily available, are the choice of seasoned professionals. Creams generally come in either a tub or tube, have a thick and tacky consistency, contain no irritating chemicals, and require water to form a lather. Shaving soaps are similar to creams but are sold in hard cakes (like bars of soap). One can rub a wet shaving brush directly on a cake of soap or shave some soap flakes into a bowl before mixing with a wet brush to create lather. Mixed properly, traditional shaving creams and soaps produce a rich, satisfying lather.

SHAVING OIL

For those wishing to further protect their skin against the scrape of the razor, shaving oils can be applied directly to the face to provide an extra layer of lubrication.

STYPTIC STICK AND ALUM BLOCK

Used to stop bleeding caused by nicks and cuts, these handy tools—available as either a short stick or block that can be applied directly to the face—are effective and are made of natural minerals.

AFTERSHAVE

Originally used as a disinfectant, alcohol-fueled aftershaves are splashed on the face to provide a cool, bracing finish to the shaving ritual, and are still the norm for most men. Updated formulas that rely on cooling oils instead of potentially harsh chemicals are readily available in most natural foods stores.

MOUSTACHE WAX

This tacky substance, which separates moustache novices from the professionals, comes in a variety of consistencies and colors. Those with wiry hair might have better luck using a stiffer wax while straighter moustaches tend to benefit from a softer variety. There are many brands available online and in specialty stores—take some for a test-drive to learn which works best for you. Tip: To remove non-water-soluble waxes, work a small amount of baby oil into the moustache before washing thoroughly with soap.

POMADE

A relative of moustache wax, pomade is often used to style both hair and moustaches. It is considerably less tacky than wax and remains greasy instead of drying firm, but works well at reining in wild hairs and providing a medium for light styling.

SHAVING MIRROR

A lighted, magnifying (possibly fogless) shaving mirror will be your greatest ally in doing the detail work involved in maintaining your moustache, not to mention for everyday shaving.

"Being kissed by a man who didn't wax his moustache was—like eating an egg without salt."

— Rudyard Kipling, *The Story of the Gadsbys*

SHAVING *and* GROOMING BASICS

Whether you're just getting your peach fuzz or simply need to brush up on the basics, these step-by-step instructions will help you to get the most out of your shave.

BEFORE THE SHAVE

☞ Growing a full beard and moustache is recommended before trying most styles. Be sure, though, to use an electric trimmer to clip any hair that is too long to shave with a razor.

☞ It's always preferable to shave after a hot shower. The heat naturally opens pores and acts to relax facial hair, allowing for a closer and more comfortable shave.

THE WET SHAVE

☞ Prepare and apply your shaving cream, gel, soap, or foam of choice. If using a shaving brush, apply the cream to your face in a circular motion. Otherwise, massage the cream into your beard using your fingers.

☞ Heat the blade of the razor under warm running water.

☞ Use your finger to draw a line in the shaving cream where you want your sideburns to end. Generally, this is just above the bottom of your ear, although some styles (and personal preferences) call for longer or shorter sideburns.

☞ Begin at the top of the cheeks, shaving in the same direction that your facial hair grows (called shaving with the grain). Shave only about 2 inches at a time, rinsing the blade under warm water after each stroke. As you move down to the neck and chin, take special care when rounding any corners of your face to minimize nicks or cuts.

☞ If another pass of the razor is needed, relather and make your second pass going against the grain of the beard hairs.

THE DRY SHAVE

A dry shave is a quick and easy alternative to a wet shave. While not as comfortable or close as a wet shave, it does make business trips or extended stays in airport hotels a little more bearable.

☞ Follow the electric razor manufacturer's instructions regarding shaving motion, making sure to apply minimum pressure to the face whenever possible.

AFTER THE SHAVE

☞ Rinse with cold water to close up facial pores. If using aftershave, pat it on with your hands and allow to air dry.

☞ If using moustache wax, allow moustache hair to remain moist. Gather a small quantity of wax between your thumb and forefinger and work gently into the moustache (see specific styles for application instructions). Wait ten to fifteen minutes for the wax to partially dry. Using your fingers, pull and twist hairs into position, and allow to dry completely.

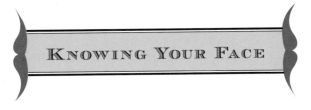

Knowing your way around your face means being able to identify key landmarks. Use these helpful illustrations to familiarize yourself with the basics:

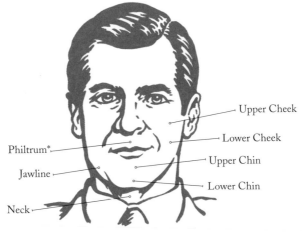

Upper Cheek

Lower Cheek

Philtrum*

Upper Chin

Jawline

Lower Chin

Neck

"What I look for mostly in a man is humor, honesty, and a moustache."

— Sally Field

*THE AREA JUST BELOW THE MIDDLE OF THE NOSE.

Moustache Styles

There's no trick to growing a 'stache—all you have to do is stop shaving. Styling a look you'll be proud of, on the other hand, takes a little know-how. Never fear, this chapter includes all the info you need to begin grooming a 'stache that is sure to win you praise (and maybe even an award).

THE NATURAL

A.K.A.: THE STASHQUATCH

WHO WORE IT: CAVEMEN,
NATURE LOVERS

TIME TO GROW: 1+ MONTHS

DIFFICULTY:

For every whiskered fellow willing to wax and snip to create a gold-medal style, there are undoubtedly ten who would rather let nature simply take its course—to beautiful effect. It's no surprise, then, that the Natural is perhaps the most ubiquitous style found throughout the world. But even in its effortlessness there's an art, albeit subtle, to the Natural moustache. Whether it's big and bushy or reserved and naturally neat, the moustache you were born with could be the best style ever.

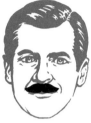

INSTRUCTIONS

Begin by shaving the cheeks, neck, and chin. Allow moustache hair to extend no more than ½ inch past the sides of the upper lip. If moustache hair in your mouth makes you uncomfortable, use moustache scissors to snip any hairs that hang below the top of the upper lip, or use a moustache comb to brush the hairs to the sides.

GROOMING

By its nature, the Natural has a tendency to grow outside the lines. Aside from shaving regularly, use moustache scissors as needed to trim unwanted or wild hairs.

VARIATIONS

The Natural doesn't stand for excessive styling. That said, it's not uncommon to see this look transformed with some fancy brushwork. For formal occasions, try taming your beast by brushing the hairs to the side. An in-a-pinch Walrus (p. 48) can also be achieved by brushing the hairs down over the lip.

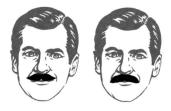

Thinking about letting your Natural 'stache grow to a record-breaking length? You've got some stiff competition—Badamsinh Juwansinh Gurjar, from western India, holds the world record with a breathtaking 12½ feet of whiskers.

HOW TO WEAR IT

Without adding a stitch, this untamed style proclaims a wearer's wild side. To really play this up, shoot for a rugged cowboy look. Boot-cut jeans and a plaid shirt look great when topped off by a leather Stetson. Taking this look to the streets is easy, too. For an urban version, go hip with skinny denim shorts, canvas shoes, and a faded monotone T-shirt.

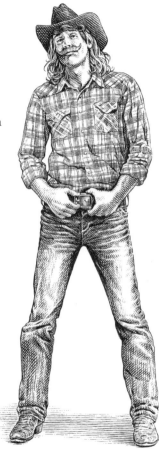

THE CRUSTACHE

A.K.A. THE NOSTACHE,
THE BARELY THERE

WHO WORE IT: YOUNG MEN OF ALL AGES

TIME TO GROW: 1+ MONTHS

DIFFICULTY:

Depending on how you look at it, the Crustache is either a real moustache or something on the way to being one. Regardless, the style's characteristically light growth, easily spotted on men coming of age, can stand alone as a badge of fully matured cool. To truly own this style, go easy on the irony and instead pay attention to nailing the subtlety of this ultra-smooth style.

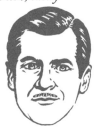

Begin by cleanly shaving cheeks, neck, and chin, allowing the upper-lip hair to extend only ½ inch past the sides of the mouth. Using moustache scissors, trim moustache hair to just above stubble length, roughly $\frac{1}{16}$ to $\frac{1}{8}$ inch. Finally, use a razor to shave just below the nose, leaving a moustache just above the upper lip.

GROOMING

Unattended, the Crustache can quickly transform into a full-blown moustache. Aside from shaving regularly, use moustache scissors frequently to keep moustache hair to appropriate shortness.

VARIATIONS

Any moustache trimmed down to the meager length of the Crustache instantly becomes a "ghost 'stache" for that style. Experiment with the Horseshoe (p. 44) or the Full Circle (p. 110) and just watch as your street cred goes through the roof.

HOW TO WEAR IT

Favored by trailer park princes, this style can go from zero to trashy in the time it takes to throw on some baggy jeans and a sleeveless T-shirt. However, as most who choose this style will undoubtedly be looking to capitalize on its edginess without looking like a fifteen-year-old, try something with unassuming class, like a pair of skinny jeans and a snug-fitting polo shirt.

A small bit of growth not only looks good on fellows—a subtle 'stache can make a bold and debatably attractive statement on women as well. Doubters need look no further than Frida Kahlo, who famously featured both her thin moustache and full eyebrows in self-portraits.

Do   Don't

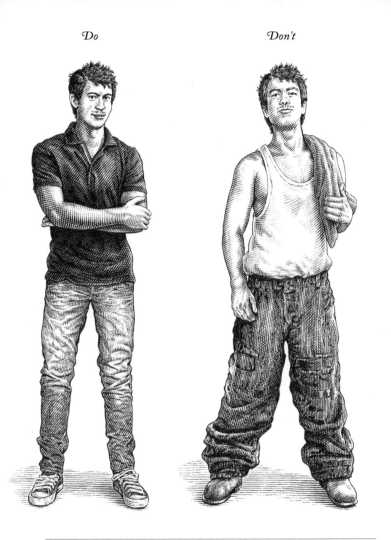

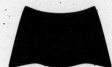

THE
TOOTHBRUSH

A.K.A.: THE CHARLIE CHAPLIN,
THE SOUL 'STACHE, THE TRAMP
WHO WORE IT: CHARLIE CHAPLIN, OLIVER HARDY,
ADOLF HITLER
TIME TO GROW: 1+ MONTHS
DIFFICULTY: 👨 👨

Subtle and sophisticated, the Toothbrush is easy to grow but somewhat difficult to pull off. Cultivating it is a cinch, making it a likely candidate for burgeoning moustachioed men. Its close association with a certain dictator, however, presents a challenge not to be undertaken by the faint of face. Paired with a carefully selected outfit, though, this classic set of whiskers can dazzle crowds just as it did before Hitler grew his infamous brush.

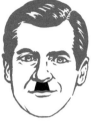

INSTRUCTIONS

Begin by cleanly shaving the cheeks, neck, and chin. Use moustache scissors to trim the bottom of the moustache, cropping the hairs to just above the upper lip. Next, use a razor to cleanly shave both sides of the moustache, leaving only a thick band of hair approximately 1 inch wide directly below the nose. Finally, use a moustache comb to brush the hair downward.

GROOMING

Aside from regular shaving, use scissors to keep the moustache hair trimmed to just above the top of the upper lip.

VARIATIONS

The Toothbrush can be styled in two distinct ways—either with straight sides or flared at the bottom. The moustache will naturally flare—to keep the sides perfectly parallel, use moustache scissors to regularly trim outlying hairs from the sides of the bottom of the moustache. Apply a small amount of moustache wax, if needed, to help the moustache keep its straight shape.

Echoing the hopes of precocious young men everywhere, Charlie Chaplin described in his autobiography how he adopted his trademark "tramp" moustache in an attempt to appear older for a film role. The short Toothbrush (which was actually made of fake crepe hair) had the added benefit of not obscuring Chaplin's facial expressions.

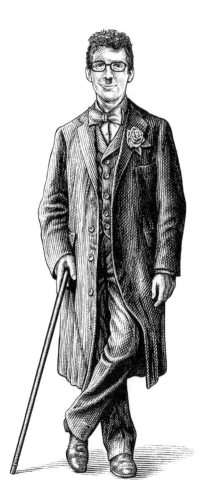

HOW TO WEAR IT

Any outfit even remotely military is, of course, out of the question. To really make the Toothbrush sing, lighten the mood by choosing clothes with a vaudevillian flair—a long dress coat, bow tie, and cane, for example. Chunky black horn-rimmed glasses echo the 'stache's bold line and add a welcome touch of nerdy sophistication.

THE CHEVRON

A.K.A.: THE MAGNUM, THE CHEVY

WHO WORE IT: TOM SELLECK, MARK SPITZ, FREDDIE MERCURY

TIME TO GROW: 1+ MONTHS

DIFFICULTY:

Ever since Tom Selleck donned a Chevron in his role as easygoing Hawaiian P.I. Thomas Magnum, the cool yet rugged look has been synonymous with boyish charm. Hanging like a shaggy inverted V over the upper lip, the Chevron is an ideal moustache for novices who might be intimidated by fancy waxes or precision detailing. Offering maximum style points with minimum upkeep, it's no wonder that the Chevron is also a popular choice among seasoned growers.

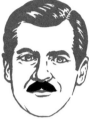

Styling a Chevron is a snap. Begin by cleanly shaving the cheeks, neck, and chin. The moustache hair should not extend more than ½ inch past the sides of the mouth. Shave the very top hairs on either side of the moustache, shaping it into a subtle inverted-V shape. Next, use trimming scissors to clip the bottom hairs so that they just hang over the top of the upper lip. Don't snip any more than you have to—the Chevron looks the best when left a little bit shaggy.

GROOMING

Aside from regular shaving and a few snips to keep wild hairs in check, the Chevron is a blissfully effortless style to maintain.

VARIATIONS

To graduate from boyish charm to ultimate tough guy, sculpt a look that blends the Chevron and the Horseshoe (p. 44). Follow the instructions above but shave only the very center of the chin, leaving a ¼-inch line of hair extending from each moustache tip to the bottom of the chin.

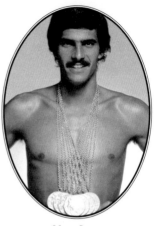

⊰MARK SPITZ⊱

"A Russian coach asked me if my moustache slowed me down. I said, 'No, as a matter of fact, it deflects water away from my mouth, allows my rear end to rise, and makes me bullet-shaped in the water, and that's what allowed me to swim so great.'"

— Mark Spitz, Olympic gold-medal swimmer

HOW TO WEAR IT

A Hawaiian shirt and shorts are all it takes to transform yourself into a Magnum-style beachcomber. Or, take a page from Freddie Mercury's book and go with a biker look complete with studded leather jacket and chaps. Whatever look you choose, a pair of mirror sunglasses is sure to pair well.

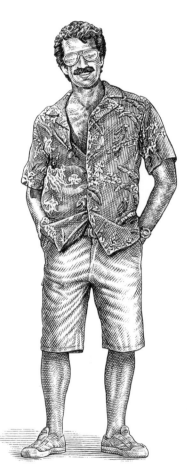

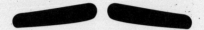

THE PENCIL

A.K.A.: THE THIN LIZZY,
THE UPPER CRUST

WHO WORE IT: JOHN WATERS, GOMEZ ADAMS,
CLARK GABLE

TIME TO GROW: 1+ MONTHS
DIFFICULTY:

Recent decades have sequestered this style to the realm of lounge lizards and Vegas hustlers, but the Pencil has historically been held as a mark of cool sophistication. Any doubters can reference Clark Gable's closely cropped whiskers in his role of Rhett Butler in Gone with the Wind. *Depending on how your wear it, this moustache—thin enough to have been traced by a pencil—is perfect for a raucous night of partying or for a swank gallery opening.*

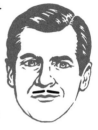

INSTRUCTIONS

Begin by cleanly shaving the cheeks, neck, and chin, leaving the upper-lip hair to extend no more than ½ inch past the sides of the mouth. Using a razor, cleanly shave directly below the nose, leaving a flat, thin line of hair approximately ¼ inch in height just above the upper lip. Finally, use moustache scissors or an electric trimmer to detail the moustache's bottom line. Be careful not to trim too short—there's a fine line between a perfectly groomed Pencil and a Crustache (p. 24).

GROOMING

Aside from regular shaving, use moustache scissors or an electric trimmer to maintain a maximum hair length of about $^1/_8$ inch.

VARIATIONS

For a more manicured and sophisticated look, separate the two sides of the moustache by using trimming scissors to cleanly clip the small amount of hair over the philtrum (p. 17). For a more caddish effect, work a very small amount of wax into the moustache, just enough to give it a glassy sheen.

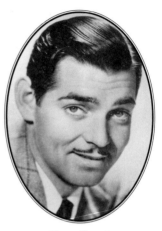

⊱CLARK GABLE⊰

Originally released as "Pencil Thin Moustache," Jimmy Buffett's 1974 song was quickly rereleased as "Pencil Thin *Mustache*," highlighting the popular confusion surrounding the word's spelling. Today, American English favors "mustache" while the British, as well most of the rest of the world (including the competitive circuit), tend toward "moustache."

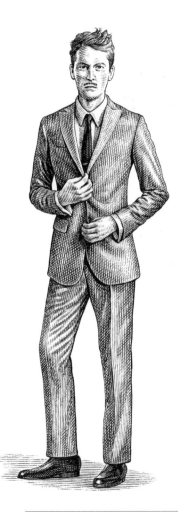

HOW TO WEAR IT

Whether you're slithering around the lounge scene or have a rendezvous with the slot machines, the Pencil is your one-way ticket to kitschy cool. Strike a relaxed pose by rocking *Miami Vice*–style white slacks and a flamboyant neon shirt. Alternatively, if you want to promote a devil-may-care sophistica-tion, sharpen your act with a tight-fitting dark suit and light-colored shirt. For added effect, sling on a razor-thin spaghetti or bolo tie.

THE PAINTER'S BRUSH

A.K.A.: THE BRUSHSTACHE,
THE AVERAGE 'MO
WHO WORE IT: BURT REYNOLDS
TIME TO GROW: 1+ MONTHS
DIFFICULTY:

Just like a wide, bristly brush is to a house painter, this unassuming style is an essential addition to any moustache aficionado's toolbox. Just covering the width of the upper lip and accented with subtly rounded corners, the Painter's Brush exists comfortably between the bushy Chevron (p. 32) and the trim Pencil (p. 36). Never showy, the Painter's Brush is the perfect look for those who crave a moustache but aren't hungry for undue attention.

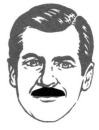

INSTRUCTIONS

Begin by cleanly shaving the cheeks, neck, and beard, leaving the upper-lip hair to extend about ½ inch past the sides of the mouth. Use trimming scissors to snip any wild hairs from the bottom of the moustache, leaving a clean, flat line just above the upper lip. To finish, use the scissors to trim the tops of the very tips of the moustache, rounding them slightly.

GROOMING

Aside from regular shaving, continue to use trimming scissors to round the top corners of each tip and maintain a clean line on the bottom of the moustache.

VARIATIONS

The Painter's Brush is a look that doesn't take well to fancy embellishments. Trim it too much and you might end up with a Chevron (p. 32); let it grow too long and you'll have a full-blown Horseshoe (p. 44)

on your hands—or your upper lip. For a subtle accentuation, though, try incorporating a small amount of moustache wax, which will add a faint but welcome shine. Another option is to make vertical snips into the moustache with a pair of moustache scissors. While this won't fundamentally change the moustache, it will provide for a more bristly brush.

If a real paintbrush is more fitting with your character, try adding a splash of color to your 'stache via store-bought hair coloring. Go green for St. Patty's Day or orange for Halloween—there's a rainbow of possibilities.

HOW TO WEAR IT

The Painter's Brush speaks to the everyman in all of us and fittingly does not need to be dressed up. A colorful, well-worn polo or other knitted shirt and comfortable slacks or chinos will transform you into the picture of unassuming moustachioed style.

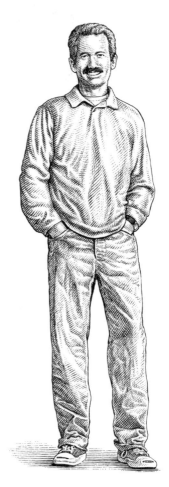

THE HORSESHOE

A.K.A: THE WRESTLER, THE LENNON

WHO WORE IT: HULK HOGAN, JOHN LENNON, SHAQUILLE O'NEAL

TIME TO GROW: 1+ MONTHS

DIFFICULTY:

For those seeking a style that will cement their place in the pantheon of manliness, look no further. This fearsome moustache begins with a full brush that hangs like a crowbar over the upper lip. Meanwhile, the ends plummet down to the bottom of the chin, framing the mouth in a horseshoe-shaped arc. Real horseshoes might bring good luck, but you won't need any of it when sporting this commanding set of whiskers.

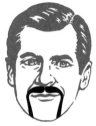

INSTRUCTIONS

Beginning with a natural beard and moustache (see the Lumberjack, p. 86), use trimming scissors or electric clippers to trim all facial hair to a length of ¼ to ½ inch. Next, use a razor to cleanly shave the chin, taking care not to shave beyond the width of the mouth. Continuing with the razor and beginning below the ears, shave both the neck and cheeks, moving progressively toward the mouth with each stroke. On each side of the face, stop when you have remaining a band of hair about ½ inch wide extending from the tips of the moustache to the base of the chin. Finally, use the razor to shave any neck hair remaining below the chin.

Aside from regular shaving, use scissors to keep any wild hairs in check.

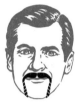

For a look that screams living on the edge, use an electric trimmer to shave a series of thin slanted lines into the hair below the mouth. Spacing each line ¼ inch apart and angling each slightly upward to the mouth, you'll be ready for any barroom brawl.

Horseshoe-moustache icon John Lennon got a little help from his friends when the Beatles all grew moustaches for the recording of their 1967 album *Sgt. Pepper's Lonely Hearts Club Band*, which originally included a cardboard moustache cutout in the record's cover sleeve.

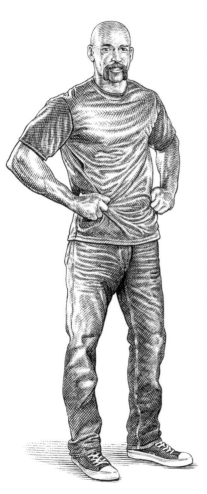

HOW TO WEAR IT

This burly yet versatile style can be dressed up in a variety of ways depending on the occasion. For an intensely macho effect, wear a tight-fitting T-shirt (wrestlers prefer a sleeveless model) paired with jeans. For dressier occasions, a combination of a dark-colored dress shirt and pants will complete a dashing rogue effect. A bolo tie, mirroring the Horseshoe's vertical lines, finishes the look.

THE WALRUS

A.K.A.: THE CRUMB CATCHER,
THE SOUP STRAINER
WHO WORE IT: FRIEDRICH NIETZSCHE,
MARK TWAIN, CHESTER A. ARTHUR
TIME TO GROW: 3+ MONTHS
DIFFICULTY:

This stately 'stache is as substantial as its namesake. Characterized by low-hanging hairs that hide most or all of the mouth, the Walrus reached a high point in popularity around the turn of the last century when it was a style of choice among high-ranking politicians and highbrow intellectuals. Today, the Walrus is a favorite among those with antiquarian tastes who don't mind a few crumbs hanging around in their 'stache.

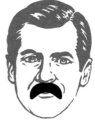

INSTRUCTIONS

Begin by cleanly shaving the cheeks, neck, and chin. The remaining hair on the upper lip should extend only about ½ inch past the sides of the mouth. Use moustache scissors to trim any wild hairs from the top of the moustache. To complete the look, use a moustache comb to brush the hairs downward to fall over the mouth. Depending on your level of tidiness, you may wish to trim a clean line along the bottom of the moustache, taking care to trim as little as possible.

GROOMING

As it grows, the Walrus will creep farther down your face as well as to the sides. Use trimming scissors whenever necessary to maintain a clean bottom line, as well as to snip any unwanted growth outward toward the cheeks.

VARIATIONS

The thick and bushy Walrus presents an open palette for creative moustache artists. Use a pair of moustache scissors to trim your moustache into long strips, mimicking the teeth in a comb. Or, apply a small amount of wax and roll the bottom of the 'stache outward, forming an upward curl.

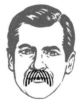

Aside from Chester A. Arthur, only two other presidents have elected to sport a 'stache sans beard: Theodore Roosevelt and William Taft.

HOW TO WEAR IT

The long, dramatic Walrus looks best when worn with an equally long dress coat and wire-rimmed glasses. For a traditional look, choose dark colors like gray or black. Or, if the style of a Southern gentleman is what you're after, a snappy white suit is just the ticket.

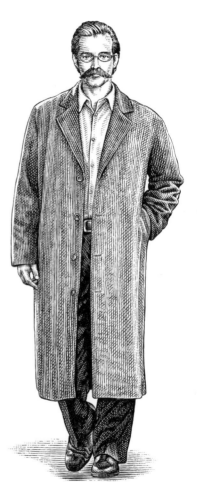

THE PYRAMID

A.K.A.: THE LAMPSHADE

WHO WORE IT: MODERN-DAY PHARAOHS

TIME TO GROW: 1+ MONTHS

DIFFICULTY:

There's something to be said for going with the flow. Unlike some moustache styles that use waxes to defy gravity, the Pyramid draws its strength from the moustache's natural shape. Anything but staid, the triangular shape allows for plenty of variation. However you shave it, though, the Pyramid will firmly mark you as a purist who isn't afraid to have a little fun.

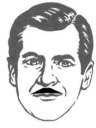

INSTRUCTIONS

Begin by cleanly shaving the cheeks, neck, and chin, allowing no upper-lip hair to extend past the sides of the mouth. Using moustache scissors, trim the moustache hairs so that they end just above the upper lip. Then use a razor to shave a thin strip just below the nose. Next, shave both sides of the moustache in a diagonal line that begins near the nose and descends toward the side of the face. Finally, shave only the very tips of the moustache to create a clean vertical line on each end.

GROOMING

Aside from regular shaving, trim the moustache hairs regularly, not allowing them to extend past the top of the upper lip.

VARIATIONS

The Pyramid is the starting point for a score of variations. Experiment by taking the same basic shape and varying the size. You can have a Petit Pyramid that falls just outside the width of the nose or a Grande Pyramid that extends outside the confines of the upper lip.

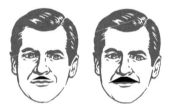

Having fun with geometric moustaches doesn't have to end with pyramids. Try shaping your 'stache into a circular shape or, for a serious challenge, use your beard and moustache together to form a hexagon.

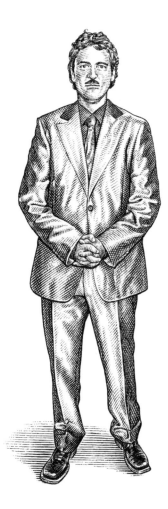

HOW TO WEAR IT

There's something pleasantly bizarre about this stylized 'stache. Use this to your advantage by choosing an outfit that really makes a statement. Maybe the best source for kooky, cool inspiration are the members of Devo, who might suggest sporting tight-fitting suits that feature metallic or highly contrasting colors. A spaghetti tie makes a nice final touch (but leave the dog-bowl hat at home).

THE FU MANCHU

A.K.A.: THE EMPEROR, THE FU TANG

WHO WORE IT: JIMI HENDRIX, FRANK BLACK, ANTON LAVEY

TIME TO GROW: 6+ MONTHS

DIFFICULTY:

Named after early twentieth-century author Sax Rohmer's devious character Dr. Fu Manchu, this moustache has become the style of choice for a century of cinematic archvillains and those seeking to cultivate a distinctively Eastern appeal. While Rohmer faced harsh criticism for his book's negative portrayal of Chinese immigrants, Fu Manchu's namesake whiskers have become a calling card for students of Eastern philosophy, martial arts fanatics, and moustache aficionados shooting for a more eccentric image.

INSTRUCTIONS

While it takes considerable time to grow, this impressive 'stache is deceptively easy to pull off. Start by cleanly shaving the cheeks, neck, and chin. Be careful not to clip off any hair from the tips of the moustache. The remaining hair on the upper lip should extend only about ½ inch down toward the sides of the mouth. Use a moustache comb to part the moustache, brushing hair from the center outward. Use a pair of moustache scissors to trim any wild or unwanted hair from the body of the moustache. If using wax, work a small amount into the moustache and wait approximately ten to fifteen minutes. Use your fingers to pull the hair at the ends of the moustache downward as far as possible.

GROOMING

This style only gets better with time. Allow the moustache tips to continue growing long while keeping the rest well trimmed.

VARIATIONS

The Fu Manchu is often paired with a similarly styled beard that is grown only on the chin and shaped into two long pieces that hang down past the neck. For a truly over-the-top look, try braiding the strands of the moustache and beard together, tying each end off with a rubber band.

HOW TO WEAR IT

Traditionalists will want to pair this distinct 'stache with a mandarin-collared shirt. For a more Westernized approach, choose a button-up shirt with a short collar and cufflinks, together with slacks and a button-up vest.

Curiously, Rohmer's original book contained no description of Fu Manchu's facial hair. The doctor's signature whiskers didn't appear until actor Warner Oland sported them in a 1929 film adaptation.

Mandarin

Western

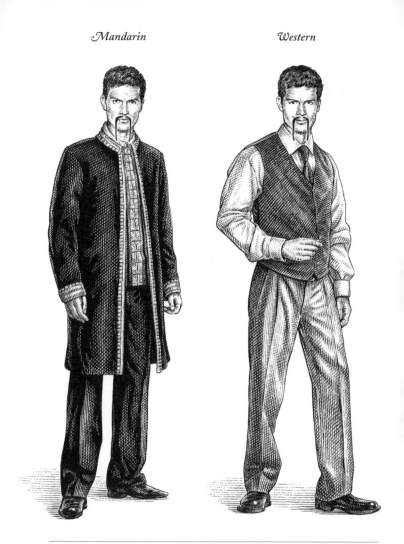

THE HANDLEBAR

A.K.A.: THE SPAGHETTI 'STACHE
WHO WORE IT: ROLLIE FINGERS,
MICHAEL "ATTERS" ATTREE
TIME TO GROW: 3+ MONTHS
DIFFICULTY:

Reminiscent of dastardly villains, British infantry, and dapper detectives, the Handlebar is perhaps the most classic of styles. This quintessential 'stache is easily recognizable by its artistically waxed tips, curving upward to mimic a pair of bicycle handlebars. Don't be fooled by this style's elegant simplicity; grooming the perfect Handlebar can be a lifelong pursuit. Just ask the members of England's prestigious Handlebar Club, who have been meeting to wax—both moustache and philosophic—since 1947.

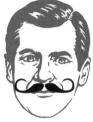

INSTRUCTIONS

Begin by cleanly shaving the cheeks, neck, and chin. The hair on your upper lip should remain full and unclipped. After moistening the moustache with a little water, use a moustache comb to part the moustache down the middle, brushing the hair from the center out toward the sides, and finally swooping down toward the chin. Next, take a small amount of moustache wax and work it into the moustache, beginning in the middle and working outward. As you reach the tips, gently curl them upward. Wait about five minutes for the wax to firm up. When the wax is firm but still pliable, use your fingers to curl the moustache tips upward and in toward the nose, stopping just short of creating a full circle with the tips.

GROOMING

Shave daily and reapply wax as needed. It might take a month or more for the moustache to naturally hold the handlebar shape, although a small amount of wax will be necessary to hold it in place.

VARIATIONS

For a Petit Handlebar à la Agatha Christie's intrepid detective Hercule Poirot, bend the waxed tips in toward the nose and then back out to create an "S" shape on either side of the nose.

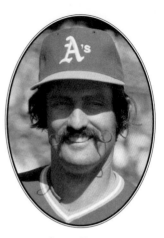

⊰Rollie Fingers⊱

Baseball legend Rollie Fingers certainly scored points with fans when he sported a luxurious Handlebar on the Oakland Athletics' opening day in 1972. While Fingers originally sprouted his whiskers as a publicity stunt, the look became so famous that he continues to wear it today.

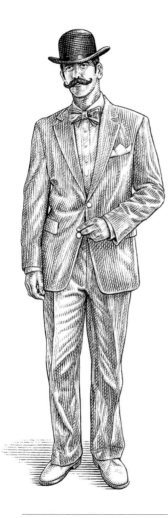

HOW TO WEAR IT

This classic moustache simply begs to be dressed up in Old English style. Try peddling around town on an antique cruiser bike while decked out in a fine tweed suit. Or, for warm summer days by the lake, opt for a tidy seersucker suit. As for accessories, you can never go wrong by pairing this look with a spiffy bowler hat and bow tie.

THE DALÍ

A.K.A.: THE SURREALIST 'STACHE,
THE PERSISTENCE OF WHISKERS
WHO WORE IT: SALVADOR DOMINGO FELIPE
JACINTO DALÍ I DOMÈNECH
TIME TO GROW: 3+ MONTHS
DIFFICULTY: 👨 👨 👨 👨 🐟

Famously flamboyant and superbly surreal, Salvador Dalí championed the idea that creativity knows no bounds. Aside from the estimated 1,500 paintings he created, perhaps the artist's most memorable stroke of genius was the signature set of whiskers that he wore for most of his life. Absurdly stylish, the Dalí blends aristocratic elegance and artistic flair to create a truly original work of art.

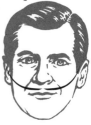

INSTRUCTIONS

Begin by cleanly shaving the cheeks, neck, and chin, leaving no upper-lip hair extending past the sides of the mouth. Next, use a moustache comb to brush the hairs from the center of the moustache outward on each side. Using moustache scissors, trim any hair on the philtrum (p. 17) as short as possible. Finally, work a small amount of wax into the moustache, beginning in the middle and working outward to the tips. Wait five to ten minutes for the wax to stiffen up. When the wax is stiff but still pliable, use your thumb and index finger to shape the ends so that they are pointing up at a steep angle, just short of vertical.

GROOMING

The dramatic effect of the Dalí is greatly increased by the length of the moustache tips. Continue regular shaving, trimming any wild hairs but allowing the tips to grow as long as possible, and reapply wax as often as needed.

VARIATIONS

The Dalí's long, moldable whiskers provide endless opportunities for creativity. A truly eye-catching look can be achieved by twirling the ends around a pencil to create spirals or curlicues.

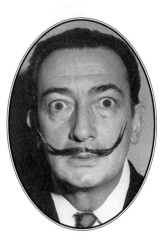

⊰Salvador Dalí⊱

One persistent, yet dubious legend about Dalí describes how, in his early years, the struggling artist used his moustache as a paintbrush to save money on supplies.

HOW TO WEAR IT

The sharp lines and glossy sheen of this style look best when coupled with an outfit that denotes refinement with a little bit of an edge. Take a page from the classy-cool Mods of the '60s by selecting trim stovepipe pants, a crisp button-down shirt, a close-fitting overcoat, and leather shoes buffed to a mirror gleam. For a dab of artistic flair, tuck a red carnation into your lapel.

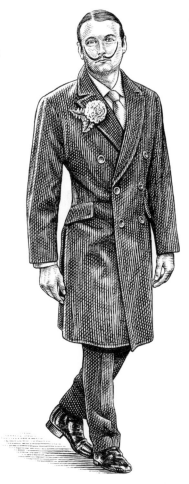

THE HUNGARIAN

A.K.A.: THE WILD WEST

WHO WORE IT: EMILIANO ZAPATA,
RESPECTABLE HUNGARIANS

TIME TO GROW: 3+ MONTHS

DIFFICULTY:

Whether it reminds you of an archduke or a frontier law-man, no one can dispute the distinct gravitas imparted by the Hungarian. Unlike the expansive Imperial style, this moustache style, famously worn by centuries of upper-class Hungarian men, uses only hair from the upper lip. That's not to say that this commanding 'stache is lacking—left unchecked, the Hungarian will soon grow into a bushy wave that washes over the face.

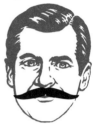

INSTRUCTIONS

Begin by cleanly shaving the cheeks, neck, and chin, leaving the hair on the upper lip to extend no more than ½ inch past the sides of the mouth. Using a moustache comb, part the moustache by brushing the hairs from the middle outward. With a pair of trimming scissors, snip any rogue hairs extending from the body of the moustache. Work a small dot of wax into the moustache's ends, pulling the hairs outward and twisting. Wait five to ten minutes for the wax to stiffen. When the wax is stiff but still pliable, use your thumb and index finger to work the ends so that they dip downward before curling back up just slightly at the tips.

GROOMING

As one of the bushiest brush styles, the Hungarian only gets better with time. Continue keeping any wild hairs in check with moustache scissors, shave regularly, and apply only as much wax as needed to keep wiry hairs together.

VARIATIONS

A more dramatic version of the Hungarian involves crossing the style with the over-the-mouth growth of the Walrus (p. 48). After a robust Hungarian has been established, gradually reduce the amount of hair you clip off the bottom section. Use a comb to pull this extra hair toward the tips so that the moustache bottom falls over both sides of the mouth. Also check out this style's championship variation, the Strongman (p. 124).

It wasn't only men of the Wild West who sported bushy 'staches. Prospectors during the gold rush of 1849 stood a good chance of losing their poker winnings to the notoriously crafty and hirsute gambler Simone Jules or, as she came to be known, Madame Moustache.

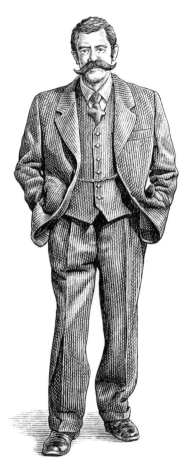

HOW TO WEAR IT

The Hungarian is a look fitting for revolutionaries and other big movers and shakers—dress accordingly. Try a rich wool suit (a three-piece will score you extra points), a shirt with a wide collar, and a thickly knotted tie. And while traditional Hungarian embroidered vests should remain in the closet, polishing off your outfit with a gold watch chain or richly patterned handkerchief is not a bad idea.

THE IMPERIAL

A.K.A.: THE ROYAL,
THE KING CUT
WHO WORE IT: KINGS AMONG MEN
TIME TO GROW: 3+ MONTHS
DIFFICULTY:

While not uniquely associated with kings, the Imperial style is grand enough for whatever royal court—or fancy dinner club—you find yourself in. Similar to its cousin the Hungarian, the Imperial is also characterized by a bushiness that is accentuated by upwardly curling ends. And to help bolster the look, the Imperial incorporates growth from the cheeks, adding support and extra body to an already dramatic, imposing brush.

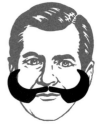

INSTRUCTIONS

Begin by cleanly shaving the chin and neck. If desired, shave only the top of the cheeks. With a moustache comb, part the moustache (including hair on the cheeks) by brushing hair from the center outward. Using a pair of trimming scissors, trim any wild hairs extending from the moustache. Work in a small dot of moustache wax, beginning at the moustache's center and moving outward. Wait five to ten minutes for the wax to become stiff yet still pliable. Use your thumb and index finger to point both ends up before curling inward toward the nose, stopping just short of a full circle.

GROOMING

Aside from regular shaving, reapply a small amount of wax each day or until your moustache becomes trained to hold its shape.

VARIATIONS

As the name suggests, the Imperial is prone to expansion. Embrace this tendency by allowing the cheek hair to completely grow out. Instead of using wax to style curls, use electric clippers to cut whatever shape you like. One popular fashion is to clip the moustache ends into thick, upwardly curling muttonchops that end in a flat, horizontal line level with the bottom of the nose.

While countless kings, dukes, and other regal characters have sported moustaches, one royal personality is conspicuously without. In a regular pack of cards, only the King of Hearts has no love for a hairy upper lip.

HOW TO WEAR IT

This grandiose style looks best when framed by outfits worthy of Hollywood's early royalty. For everyday wear, choose dapper linen suits paired with an ascot. Or, for a night on the town, opt for a black tie—and don't forget the tails.

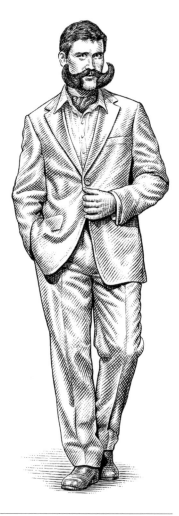

THE ENGLISH

A.K.A.: THE SIDESWIPE, THE VILLAIN
WHO WORE IT: ENLIGHTENED ENGLISHMEN,
DASTARDLY KNAVES
TIME TO GROW: 3+ MONTHS
DIFFICULTY:

The English have a habit of going big—big empires, big clocks, and even big whiskers. Featuring a neatly combed moustache extending into long waxed whiskers that stretch out horizontally like the London Bridge, the English 'stache is not to be underestimated. Loosen up your waxing fingers and get ready to twist; this style requires some serious time, determination, and a little bit of English sensibility.

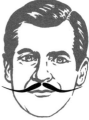

Begin by cleanly shaving the cheeks, neck, and chin, allowing the upper-lip hairs to extend only ½ inch past the sides of the mouth. Wet the moustache and use a moustache comb to part it, combing hairs from the center out toward the sides. Work a small amount of wax into the hairs, wait ten to fifteen minutes, and use your thumb and index finger to twist and pull the tips out to the side. Apply more wax, if needed, and reshape so that the whiskers stand horizontally, pointing just a bit upward, without additional support.

GROOMING

Aside from shaving regularly, reapply wax as often as needed and use scissors to snip any uneven or wild hairs from the moustache tips.

VARIATIONS

With its long, pliable ends,the English is a perfect starting point for creative growers. Let your imagination run wild as you bend and wax creative shapes. For special occasions or holidays, try shaping the ends into specific objects such as hearts or four-leaf clovers.

Long seen as a mark of masculine virility, the moustache has also been closely tied to the military throughout English history. Most notably, both the Napoleonic and Crimean Wars saw soldiers return with bushy whiskers, which sparked an explosive rise in the popularity of manly moustaches.

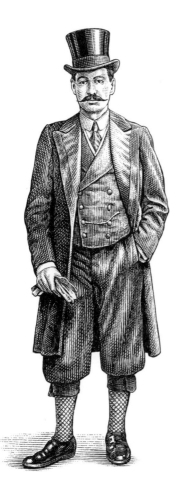

HOW TO WEAR IT

Always impressive, proper English men's attire is relatively easy to achieve. A top hat alone gets you halfway there. Knicker-bockers will win you points with traditionalists, but a tweed suit or nifty three-piece (in royal blue) will bring you up to date with impeccable style.

THE MARIO

A.K.A.: THE 8-BIT, THE RADISH 'STACHE
WHO WORE IT: MARIO THE PLUMBER
TIME TO GROW: 3+ MONTHS
DIFFICULTY:

You don't have to lurk around barbershops to catch a glimpse of one of the world's most intriguing moustaches—just play a video game. Since taking his first jump in 1981, Mario has been synonymous with malicious mushrooms, grumpy gorillas, and one super 'stache. While mastering this style will certainly prove useful for your next Halloween costume, the Mario can also be worn to add a splash of childhood fun to the starchy world of grown-ups.

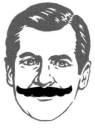

INSTRUCTIONS

Begin by cleanly shaving the cheeks, neck, and chin, allowing the upper-lip hair to extend up to an inch past the sides of the mouth. Use a moustache comb to part the moustache, brushing the hairs from the center out toward the sides. Work a liberal amount of wax into the moustache, press the moustache hairs flat, facing out, and flaring up toward the ears. Wait ten to fifteen minutes and then use your fingers to shape a scalloped edge on the bottom of the moustache.

GROOMING

This entertaining style is difficult to maintain in the long term and best used as a one-time style before shaving the 'stache into a more subtle style. If longevity is your goal, though, reapply wax and reshape as often as necessary.

VARIATIONS

While this character-specific style doesn't translate well into alternative forms, there are a vast array of characters that also sported animated whiskers. Pick your favorite and use it as an excuse to put your imagination and skills to the test.

Mario isn't the only famously moustachioed cartoon character. Here are just a few of the legions of illustrated whisker wearers:

- Wario
- Ned Flanders
- Luigi
- Yosemite Sam
- Snidely Whiplash
- Dick Dastardly

HOW TO WEAR IT

There's only one way to wear the Mario: a red T-shirt coupled with form-fitting blue overalls. A small red hat and, if available, white gloves complete the look.

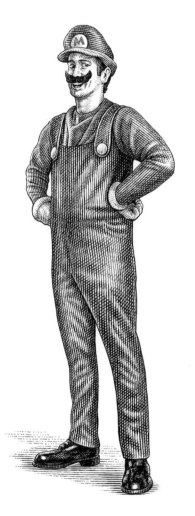

Moustache Combos

Despite their undisputable superiority, even moustaches get lonely sometimes. Luckily, there are sideburns, goatees, soul patches, and beards to keep a lonesome 'stache company. Let your hair and imagination run wild as you work your way through these fantastically furry combo styles.

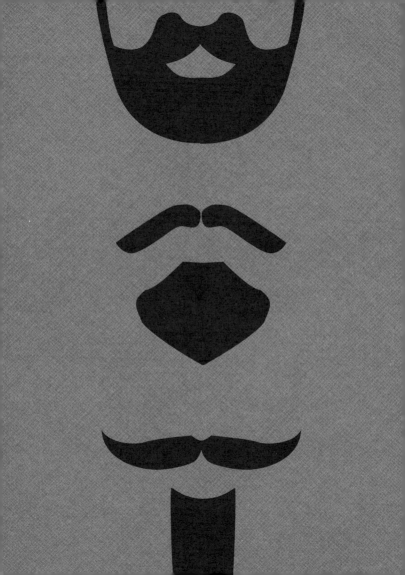

THE
LUMBERJACK

A.K.A.: THE BIG ONE, THE WILD STYLE

WHO WORE IT: PAUL BUNYAN,
ZACH GALIFIANAKIS

TIME TO GROW: 3+ MONTHS

DIFFICULTY:

When you live and work in the middle of the forest, probably the only things that are going to notice your unkempt facial hair are the squirrels. Perhaps that's why lumberjacks, both fictional and real, have become closely associated with this fuzzy style, which boasts a bushy and natural moustache and beard. Whatever the reason, the Lumberjack's effortless upkeep and aura of simpler times surely figures largely into why this look has become a favorite among thoroughly modern men. It also make a great starting point for more advanced styles— just remember to exchange your ax for a razor before shaving.

INSTRUCTIONS

This effortless style is exactly that—effortless. Simply stop shaving, allow all facial hair to grow unimpeded, and groom as often as desired. The secret to keeping this style (or any facial hair style, for that matter) looking beautiful is to keep yourself as healthy and stress-free as possible. The better you take care of your body, the better, healthier, and fuller your beard and moustache will be, too.

GROOMING

If you must, use moustache scissors to trim any moustache hair that finds its way into your mouth. Likewise, feel free to trim any beard hairs that become unwieldy or annoying.

VARIATIONS

The Lumberjack offers plenty of raw material for sculpting into whatever shape you desire. Use Tolkien as your inspiration and create a Middle-Earth masterpiece by splitting the beard into two parts and twisting each into a French braid, dwarf-style. Or, shave the upper-lip hair as well as the chin and cheeks down to the top of the jawline for a rocking Alaskan Whaler look.

Natural beard icon and former Cuban leader Fidel Castro once claimed that his impressive set of whiskers wasn't meant to be stylish; rather it was a time-saving strategy. In the book *Fidel Castro: My Life* he explains, "If you multiply the fifteen minutes you spend shaving every day by the number of days in a year, you'll see that you devote almost 5,500 minutes to shaving."

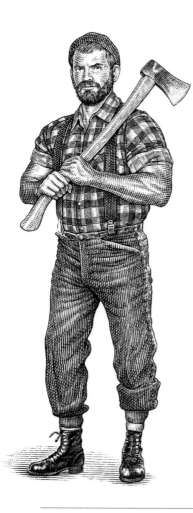

HOW TO WEAR IT

As the name implies, the Lumberjack is a style that looks best when dressed in hip, outdoorsy garb. Flannel shirts and overalls are a classic. Alternatively, if you're trying to represent a more refined nature, try a loose-fitting linen suit and shirt with a straight collar and no tie as a counterpoint to this extra-large style.

THE
BUFFALO BILL

A.K.A.: THE BILLY GOAT

WHO WORE IT: WILLIAM FREDERICK
"BUFFALO BILL" CODY

TIME TO GROW: 3+ MONTHS

DIFFICULTY:

Whether hunting on the Great Plains or entertaining European dignitaries with his traveling show, Buffalo Bill epitomized the fearless spirit of the Wild West. As a lasting legacy, his signature beard and moustache combo continues to impart frontier gentility to today's aspiring cowboys, urban or otherwise. With its unrefined set of whiskers and grizzly chin beard, the Buffalo Bill is easy to groom and looks best when allowed to grow a little wild.

Moustache: Cleanly shave the cheeks, leaving the upper-lip hair to extend only ½ inch past the sides of the mouth, taking care not to trim the tips. Use a moustache comb to part the moustache down the middle, combing hairs from the center toward the sides.

Beard: Cleanly shave the sides of the face and neck, beginning at the bottom of the sideburns. Leave unshaven a 2-inch vertical band of hair in the middle of the chin. Finally, use a comb to brush the beard hair downward so that it hangs below the chin.

GROOMING

Aside from regular shaving, use a moustache comb to part the moustache at least once a day. Likewise, use a comb to brush the beard hair downward as often as necessary.

VARIATIONS

The standard form of this style brings to mind a cowboy with other things on his mind than impeccable grooming. Still, for a somewhat citified variation try working a little wax into the moustache hairs and curling them up à la a Handlebar moustache (p. 60).

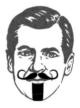

While one moustachioed Bill hunted Buffalo, another was making a name for himself as a steely-eyed lawman. Perhaps the originator of the mythological moustachioed sheriff, James Butler "Wild Bill" Hickok kept an expectedly wild set of whiskers. Unlike his contemporary, though, he kept his chin as clean as the barrel of his six-shooter.

HOW TO WEAR IT

The Buffalo Bill calls for some serious Wild West flare. Don't be scared to slip into some tight-fitting, starchy blue jeans and a handsome cotton shirt. Leather boots and even a leather hat also add a nice bit of rustic authenticity to this gallant style.

THE SHAKESPEARE

A.K.A.: THE STRATFORD-ON-LIP,
THE BARD'S BRUSH

WHO WORE IT: WILLIAM SHAKESPEARE

TIME TO GROW: 1+ MONTHS

DIFFICULTY:

Foppery aside, Elizabethan England was no stranger to good style, and no one epitomizes the period more than William Shakespeare. Aside from penning dozens of the world's most enduring and beloved plays, the Bard also found time to groom a truly dramatic set of whiskers. With its tight moustache and beard that appears as a flourish on an otherwise clean chin, the Shakespeare transforms modern wearers into timeless romantics who are all too happy to push their whiskers onto center stage.

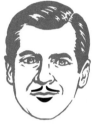

INSTRUCTIONS

Moustache: Cleanly shave the cheeks, allowing the upper-lip hair to extend only ½ inch past the sides of the mouth. Use moustache scissors to trim all moustache hair to a length between ⅛ and ¼ inch long. Part the moustache down the center by using a moustache comb to brush the hairs from the center out toward the sides. Use the scissors again to cleanly snip the hair from the philtrum (p. 17).

Beard: Cleanly shave the sides of the face and neck, begin-ning at the bottom of the sideburns. Below the mouth, leave only the soul patch (the spot of hair just beneath the lower lip) unshaven, with the hair trimmed to a length between ½ and 1 inch long. Use a comb to brush the hair downward or, for a more dramatic effect, use your fingers to twist the beard down into an upside-down triangle.

GROOMING

Aside from shaving regularly, continue to trim the moustache and beard hairs to maintain a proper length.

VARIATIONS

For a more roguish and dramatic look, continue to keep a neatly trimmed moustache but allow the beard to grow longer while maintaining its triangular shape.

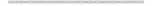

"He that hath a beard is more than a youth, and he that hath no beard is less than a man."

— *Much Ado about Nothing.* Act II, Scene 1

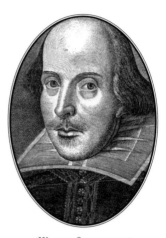

❧WILLIAM SHAKESPEARE❧

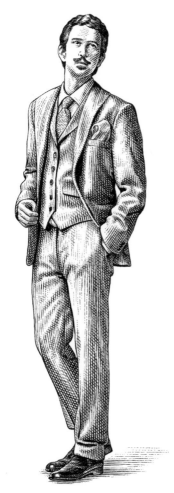

HOW TO WEAR IT

Shakespeare was an unassuming genius. Follow his lead by not overdoing this subtle yet dashing look. Fine cotton or linen suits in muted colors will ensure an appearance that's not overly dramatic and create a perfect backdrop for adding vivid accents like a colorful pocket handkerchief or patterned tie.

THE BARBER-SHOP SPECIAL

A.K.A.: THE QUARTET, THE A CAPPELLA
WHO WORE IT: WELL-GROOMED CROONERS
TIME TO GROW: 3+ MONTHS
DIFFICULTY:

Mention a barbershop quartet and what immediately springs to mind—other than melodious a cappella harmonies—are straight-brimmed hats, striped vests, bushy beards, and naturally curly moustaches. While facial hair certainly isn't a prerequisite for joining a quartet (a fact made clear by the equally popular all-female "beauty shop quartets"), this iconic look is certain to add a touch of timeless class to any fellow.

INSTRUCTIONS

Moustache: Cleanly shave the top of the cheeks, stopping at a point level to the mouth. Allow the upper-lip hair to extend only ½ inch past the sides of the mouth. Using your fingers, twist the moustache ends into an upward curl. If needed, apply water or work a very small amount of wax into the moustache before curling.

Beard: Using a comb, brush beard hair outward so that the hair flares out around the face. Snip any wild hairs with a pair of moustache scissors. The final beard should form a consistent band around the face and have a hair length of between 1 and 2 inches on the chin and between ½ and 1 inch just below the sideburns.

GROOMING

Aside from regular shaving, use a pair of trimming scissors to keep any wild hair in check and apply either water or wax to the moustache for curling purposes as often as needed.

VARIATION

This singsong style is a great starting point for experimentation. One of the easiest departures is to use a razor to shave the chin, leaving all other hair the same, for a dramatic and bristly interpretation of the Burnside (p. 118).

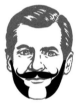

Aside from trimming hair, beards, and moustaches, medieval barbers also commonly practiced dentistry and surgery. In fact, the red and white barber's pole of today represents the bandages used in bloodletting that were hung to dry outside of a barber's shop.

HOW TO WEAR IT

Traditional quartet style mandates a colorfully striped vest, button-down shirt, slacks, and a flat-brimmed straw hat. If you're searching for a more refined look, opt for the same outfit sans the hat and with the addition of a gold watch chain or wire-rimmed glasses.

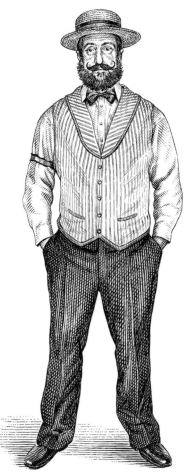

THE AERONAUT

A.K.A.: THE MAGICIAN'S ASSISTANT
WHO WORE IT: AERONAUT CAPTAINS,
MAGICIANS, TIME TRAVELERS
TIME TO GROW: 3+ MONTHS
DIFFICULTY:

This style would feel right at home on the face of a steam-powered dirigible pilot soaring among the clouds. Even if your aspirations aren't so lofty, you can still add a little industrial-age magic to your every day with this whimsical style. Combining a dapper Verdi beard (p. 108) and a dramatically curly Handlebar-style moustache (p. 60), the Aeronaut blends Victorian refinement with a daredevil sense of adventure.

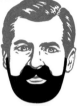

INSTRUCTIONS

Moustache: Cleanly shave the cheeks, leaving the upper-lip hair to extend only ½ inch past the sides of the mouth. Using a moustache comb, comb hairs from the center to the sides. Work a small amount of moustache wax into the hair, allow to dry for ten to fifteen minutes, and then use thumb and index finger to curve the ends downward before swooping them back up in a partial curl.

Beard: Cleanly shave the tops of the cheeks. Use trimming scissors or electric trimmers to shorten the hairs on the edges of the beard while leaving the hairs in the center long, creating a subtle cone shape on the chin. Use a razor to cleanly shave any stray hairs from the neck, creating a clean line at the bottom of the beard.

GROOMING

Aside from regular shaving, reapply wax as often as needed. You can also apply a small amount of pomade to your beard to give it a complementary shine.

VARIATIONS

Take this style to the limit by splitting the beard into two vertical tufts of hair and using a small amount of pomade to shape the sides into a pair of upturned points flaring out to the sides.

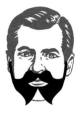

One of the most curious moustache accessories popularized during the Victorian era was cups that allowed moustachioed men to sip beverages without fear of drowning their whiskers. Called moustache cups, these handy ceramics featured a small interior ledge that protected the moustache while liquid flowed through a small opening in the base of the ledge.

HOW TO WEAR IT

The Aeronaut is no slouch when it comes to whimsy and fun. Dress it up in your finest tuxedo, nautical gear, or bomber pilot outfit—extra points for any turn-of-the-century accessories such as a monocle, pocket watch, or pipe.

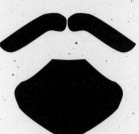

THE LENIN

A.K.A.: THE MUSTASHKY,
THE RED 'STACHE
WHO WORE IT: VLADIMIR LENIN
TIME TO GROW: 3+ MONTHS
DIFFICULTY: 🥸 🥸 🥸

Dictators come and go, but good style is eternal. Lenin surely had a similar thought each morning as he stood in front of the sink and shaved his signature faci (p.108) al hairstyle. Combining a tapered version of the Verdi beard with a well-kept, unassuming moustache, this look lends its wearer an air of stern self-confidence. Given that it was able to both inspire and strike fear into the hearts of millions, the Lenin is an excellent style to test drive at your next business conference.

INSTRUCTIONS

Moustache: Cleanly shave the cheeks and neck, leaving unshaven a circle of hair that fully encompasses the chin and allows the upper-lip hair to extend no more than ½ inch past the sides of the mouth. Using moustache scissors, trim the moustache hair, including the tips, to a length of approximately ¼ inch. Use a razor to shave the area beneath the nose, leaving only a ¼- to ½-inch strip of hair just above the upper lip.

Beard: Using trimming scissors, shape the beard hair into a rounded point with the shortest hairs around the longer hair, approximately 3 inches long, in the center. Use a razor to cleanly shave the areas just to the sides of the mouth, creating a gap between the ends of the moustache and the beard, as well as the soul patch.

GROOMING

Aside from regular shaving, use moustache scissors to keep the moustache hairs trimmed and the beard shaped to a rounded point.

VARIATIONS

To create a truly devilish look, heat things up by working a little pomade into the beard hair or using hair spray to curve the point of the beard up into a partial, outward-facing curl.

Named after Italian composer Giuseppe Verdi, the Verdi beard is commonly considered one that is connected to a full moustache, is relatively short, and has a rounded bottom. Variations on the style, such as the Lenin, are seemingly endless.

HOW TO WEAR IT

A pointed beard has a tendency to make the wearer appear devilish. If you wish to further cultivate this image, dress in sharply tailored, dark suits with crisp lines. For a kinder look—and one that echoes Lenin's own prerevolutionary style—opt instead for a loose cotton button-up shirt, suspenders, and comfortable wool pants.

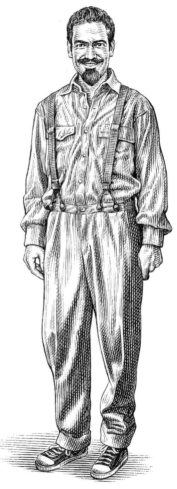

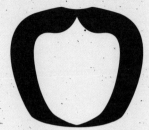

THE FULL CIRCLE

A.K.A.: THE AROUND THE WORLD
WHO WORE IT: WORLD TRAVELERS
TIME TO GROW: 3+ MONTHS
DIFFICULTY:

With moustaches, sometimes what goes around comes around. This is certainly true of the Full Circle, a circular style that bridges the gap between moustache and beard. What truly sets the Full Circle apart, though, is the exquisite definition provided via cleanly shaven cheeks and neck. The centrally framed hoop of hair that remains becomes a focal point for a look that you can dress up in myriad ways.

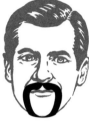

INSTRUCTIONS

Moustache: Cleanly shave the cheeks, leaving the upper-lip hair to extend only ½ inch past the sides of the mouth and taking care not to trim the tips. Use moustache scissors to snip any hair hanging down over the top lip.

Beard: Cleanly shave the sides of the face, beginning at the bottom of the sideburns. Shave the small soul patch as well as most of the hair on the chin, leaving only a thin band of hair connecting the two sides at the very bottom of the chin. Round the sides and bottom of the beard using a razor, taking care not to shave off any more hair than is necessary.

GROOMING

Aside from regular shaving, use moustache scissors to snip any moustache hair that grows over the top of the upper lip.

VARIATIONS

For a fun challenge, try trimming the Full Circle's band of hair to as fine a line as possible. Be careful, however, that you don't overdo it and snip a hole in your hoop.

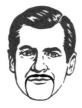

Just like the Full Circle, moustaches go all around the world. While some sources claim up to ten million American men wear whiskers, that figure pales in comparison to the estimated 80 percent of men in southern India who sport a 'stache.

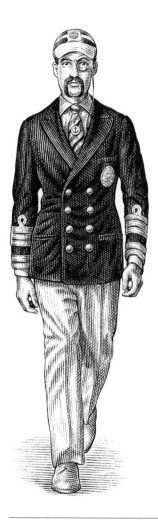

HOW TO WEAR IT

This style is an equally effective accessory to formal and fun outfits. To take it to the office or a fancy party, choose rich, woolly suits that highlight this combo's warm and bushy nature. Or, mimic the sea-savvy of a ship's captain by dressing it up nautical style—a navy-blue blazer with gold cording and an aquatic-themed tie. Peppering your outfit with circular accessories— like wire-rimmed glasses, a monocle, or a hoop earring—is a big plus.

THE MUSKETEER

A.K.A.: THE DUMAS 'DO, THE SWORDSMAN

WHO WORE IT: CYRANO DE BERGERAC; ATHOS, POR-THOS, AND ARAMIS (THE THREE MUSKETEERS)

TIME TO GROW: 3+ MONTHS

DIFFICULTY:

When nineteenth-century author Alexandre Dumas penned his story of the crafty and carousing Three Musketeers, he likely was unaware that aside from the annals of literature (and candy bars), his characters would also be forever enshrined in the moustache hall of fame. No longer appropriate only for costume parties, the Musketeer can be dressed up to add a fun spin on any occasion. Don't be intimidated by this style's rapier-sharp moustache and equally pointy goatee—the Musketeer is just a few razor strokes away from the classic English (p. 76).

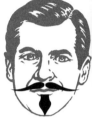

Moustache: Cleanly shave the cheeks, leaving the upper-lip hair to extend only ½ inch past the sides of the mouth. Use a moustache comb to part the moustache down the middle, combing hairs from the center toward the sides. Work a small amount of moustache wax into the hair, allow to dry for ten to fifteen minutes, and then pull the tip hairs horizontally to the side, bending the tips slightly upward.

Beard: Cleanly shave the sides of the face and the entire neck. Leave unshaven both the soul patch and a 2-inch-wide block of hair on the chin. Use your fingers to twist the beard down and into an upside-down triangle. Alternatively, use a small amount of pomade to keep the hairs together and create a finer point.

GROOMING

Aside from shaving regularly, reapply wax and/or pomade as often as needed.

VARIATIONS

A common variation on this sharp style calls for twisting and shaping the soul patch into a separate, smaller triangle that hangs just above the larger one created by the beard.

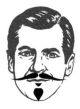

Although the title characters of Alexandre Dumas's classic novel sported eye-catching moustache styles, the author himself chose a more subtle 'stache, falling somewhere between a Chevron (p. 32) and a Walrus (p. 48).

HOW TO WEAR IT

The real musketeers were masters of seventeenth-century finery. Without looking like you shopped at a costume store, do err toward more continental attire—three-piece suits, striped ties, and bowler hats all can be mixed and matched for superb results.

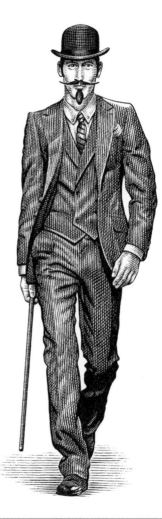

THE BURNSIDE

A.K.A.: SIDE 'STACHE, THE AFTERBURNER

WHO WORE IT: GENERAL AMBROSE

E. BURNSIDE, EMPEROR FRANZ JOSEF

OF AUSTRIA

TIME TO GROW: 3+ MONTHS

DIFFICULTY:

Despite a résumé that includes such titles as senator, governor, and U.S. Army general, Ambrose E. Burnside has a legacy that has been overshadowed by his legendary and eponymous pair of muttonchops. This look—featuring thickly sculpted sideburns connected by a wooly moustache—has the ability to transform its wearer into a formidable captain of industry sporting a luxuriant fur-lined collar.

Begin by cleanly shaving any loose hairs from the top of each cheek, taking care not to cut into the sideburns. Cleanly shave the chin to a width equal to that of the mouth. Next, pull the razor across the neck in a wide arc, beginning below the ear and cutting a line just beneath the jawline. Finally, use trimming scissors to smooth out any sharp angles to create a smooth and flowing swoop from the top of each sideburn to the tips of the moustache.

GROOMING

Shave exposed areas of the face daily to maintain a high definition. Meanwhile, use trimming scissors to keep any wild hairs in check and ensure a consistent hair length across the moustache and sideburns, separately.

VARIATIONS

The Burnside can also form the basis of a continuous loop that wraps around the entire head. Using an electric trimmer, shave a line beginning at the top of one ear and running down and around the back of the head to end at the top of the other ear. Leave a space of about 1 inch between the shaved line and the hairline.

Aside from moustaches and beards, sideburns are an entirely separate class of facial hair ripe for your exploration. Use the techniques offered in this book to create sideburn styles all your own, whether big and beefy or petit and refined.

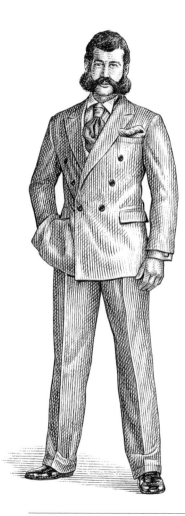

HOW TO WEAR IT

In keeping with both era and social status, this style's namesake favored a regal double-breasted suit. Opt for wide ties in bold, solid colors tied in a thick Windsor knot. A wide-collared shirt works best for everyday wear, although dandies and steampunks might revel in a more antiquarian upturned collar.

Championship Styles

You've shaved, waxed, twirled, and styled your way to the top of the moustache class. Think you're ready for the big time? Prepare yourself with these exclusive styles and tips given by some of the leaders in the field of competitive moustache growing.

THE STRONGMAN

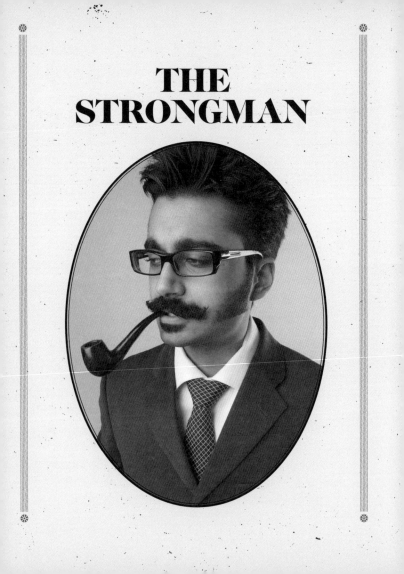

BY AMIT KUMAR
TIME TO GROW: 3+ MONTHS
DIFFICULTY: 3½

Amit Kumar, a New York–based Web software engineer, hadn't planned on growing a 'stache until he heard about the 2009 Extremely Hungary Extremely Mustache Contest, sponsored by the Hungarian Cultural Center in New York. The grand prize was especially tempting—two tickets to Budapest, Hungary. A few months and a few dabs of moustache wax later, Amit and his winning moustache— a sculpted Hungarian coupled with faded sideburns and small patch of beard—were on their way to the homeland of Hungarian 'staches, proving that even a moustache novice can become a champion.

Moustache: Begin by cleanly shaving the neck. Leave the sideburns and cheeks unshaven while allowing only ½ inch of upper-lip hair to extend past the sides of the mouth. Use a moustache comb to part the moustache by brushing the hairs from the center out toward the sides. Gather the hairs at the end of the moustache and snip the tips with scissors, cutting upward and outward in a diagonal line. Work a small amount of wax into the moustache, wait ten to fifteen minutes, and then use your thumb and index finger to work the hairs into a curl coming upward and in toward the nose.

Beard: Shave the chin, leaving only a small patch of hair directly beneath the soul patch.

Sideburns: Using an electric trimmer with a ⅛-inch attachment, shave the sideburns and cheeks. Then use a razor to further shave the cheeks, leaving a swoosh of hair extending from the sideburns to about halfway down the cheeks. Remove the attachment from the trimmer and trim the sideburn and cheek hair so that the hairs become gradually shorter as you move down from the sideburns and fade out to almost invisible stubble.

GROOMING

Aside from regular shaving, use an electric trimmer to touch up the sideburns at least once every two days and reapply moustache wax as often as necessary.

HOW TO WEAR IT

To dress up his signature style, Amit opts for a timeless gray suit, crisp white shirt, and patterned tie. If you have a pair of chunky glasses, wear them, and be sure to pick up a pipe to puff on before stepping out for the night.

"Every man should grow a moustache at least once in his life. It lets him know what he's made of."

— Amit Kumar

THE SPECIAL DELIVERY

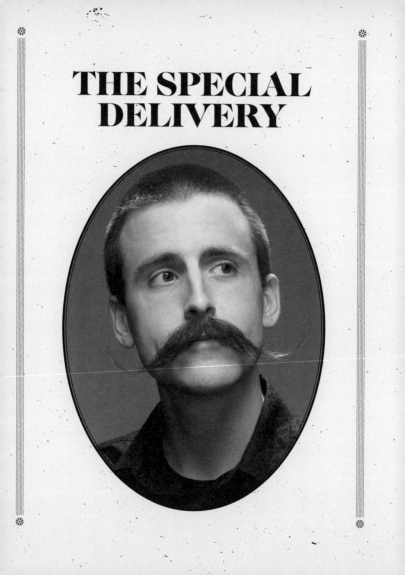

BY BEN DAVIDSON
MONTHS TO GROW: 6+
DIFFICULTY: 3½

Ben Davidson's jovial and easygoing demeanor gives few hints that he is in fact a rising star in the world of competitive moustaches. The young mailman from Ridley Park, Pennsylvania, does wear one giveaway clue just below his nose—a pristinely coiffed moustache. Davidson's natural, no-wax whiskers have won him top spots in the New York City Beard and Moustache Championships and the Coney Island Beard and Moustache Competition, as well as third place in the Natural Moustache category at the 2009 World Beard and Moustache Championships. With nothing more than hair clips, nimble fingers, and some simple tricks, Davidson sculpts an organic style that resembles a Natural Handlebar and proves that any 'stache can make a big impression with little fuss.

Begin by cleanly shaving the cheeks, neck, and chin. Leave only about ½ inch of hair extending past the edges of the mouth. Be sure not to shave off the moustache tips, which should be allowed to grow long. After a warm shower, part the moustache with your fingers and clip each side straight with a long, skinny hair clip. Wait five minutes. Remove the hair clips and use your fingers to gently twist the moustache ends into a subtle upward curl while letting the base of the moustache fall down over the upper lip. Work a small amount of hair moisturizer into the moustache, making sure to rein in any wild hairs. If desired, work a small amount of nontoxic school glue into the very tips of the moustache to help them stick together and stand slightly rigid.

GROOMING

One of Davidson's principal tricks is keeping the moustache hairs soft and supple. Aside from regularly shampooing his whiskers, he also uses an aloe vera–based shampoo every few days to give an extra dose of moisturizing. To keep the moustache growth in check, use scissors to snip as little hair as possible—as Davidson explains, "like pruning a hedge."

HOW TO WEAR IT

In contrast to moustachioed men who opt for early twentieth-century garb, Davidson uses his wardrobe to bring the moustache into the modern day. To complement this carefree yet plush 'stache, choose dark-colored shirts and slacks accentuated by a thin, metallic-colored tie. To really bring the ensemble up to speed, add an informal element like a stylish track jacket to the mix.

> "What makes a man strange enough to want to wear a giant moustache on his face? I don't know."
> — Ben Davidson

THE LASER LOOP

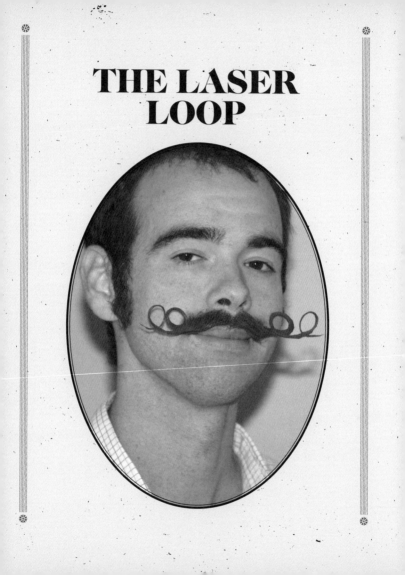

BY SAM HOLCOMBE
TIME TO GROW: 3+ MONTHS
DIFFICULTY: 4

Sam Holcombe clearly remembers the last day he shaved his moustache: May 2, 2007. That year he was set on competing in the World Beard and Moustache Championships in London, but the feeling that his moustache wasn't quite ready kept him at home in Jacksonville, Florida. So when the 2009 competition rolled around, this time in Anchorage, Alaska, the cook from the Sunshine State was ready. Along with his twin brother Devon (p. 140), he set a northern course, and returned as the third-place winner in the English Moustache category. While the English is one of Holcombe's favorites, he's also no stranger to more experimental styles, like this loopy invention inspired by a roller coaster of that name, which Sam recalls from his childhood.

Begin by cleanly shaving the cheeks, neck, and chin, allowing little to no upper-lip hair to extend past the sides of the mouth. Work a small amount of moustache wax into the hairs and wait ten to fifteen minutes. When the wax is firm yet still pliable, use your thumb and index finger to twist the hairs up and outward, forming a series of small curls on each side. If needed, apply more moustache wax and continue twisting.

GROOMING

This curly style requires a good deal of regular maintenance, not to mention moustache wax. Aside from regular shaving, reapply wax and shape moustache as often as needed.

HOW TO WEAR IT

A cook by trade, Sam scored points at the 2009 competition by sporting a starchy white chef's coat. While kitchen attire might not work for every occasion, Sam admits that keeping a moustache compels him to dress "nicer than I normally would." In that spirit, try dressing up in something casually refined—a button-up shirt and slacks, paired with a bow tie—to balance out this loopy style.

"A moustache says that you like a lot of attention. If you're a shy person, it's probably not the best thing to have."

— Sam Holcombe

THE CAT'S WHISKERS

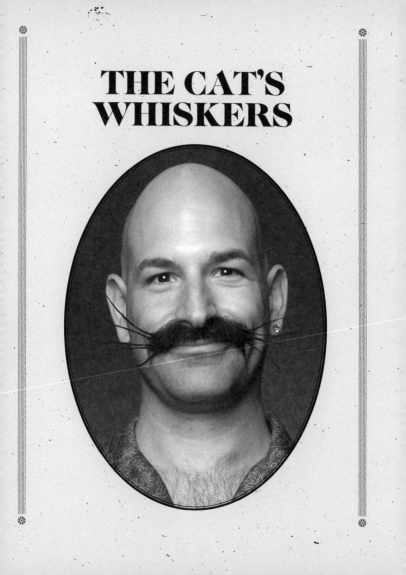

BY GANDHI JONES
TIME TO GROW: 4+ MONTHS
DIFFICULTY: 4

Gandhi Jones is a man of a thousand faces. The Seattle-based Jones (real name Keith J. Haubrich) uses his moustache as a prop in an array of elaborate alter egos, including German biker cop Herr SchwantzKopf and French gourmand Jean-Pierre Beaujolais. Jones is easy to spot on the moustache competition circuit though, where his nimble whiskers have taken top prize in such competitions as the 2009 World Beard and Moustache Championships, where he upheld his title by styling a fork-and-spoon 'stache. This look, which won Jones first place in the Freestyle Moustache category at the 2007 world championships, features long, waxy whiskers to create a look that's truly the cat's meow.

Shave the cheeks, neck, and chin. On the upper lip, leave about ½ inch of hair extending past the sides of the mouth. Use a fine-toothed comb to part the moustache, brushing hairs from the center out toward the tips. Separate each end of the moustache into five even tufts of hair. Take a small amount of wax between your thumb and index finger and work it into the separated tufts, pulling the top strands up, the bottom strands down, and the middle strands out to the side. Use small scissors to trim any unruly hairs that curl up at the ends. Wait five to ten minutes for the wax to become firm yet pliable. Use your fingers to pinch stray hairs down one last time on each whisker and arrange each in its correct position.

GROOMING

Aside from regular shaving, reapply wax and use your fingers to keep the strands separated as often as needed. Rinse wax out in warm water before going to bed.

HOW TO WEAR IT

During competitions, Jones makes sure to transform into a character that complements his whiskers. If it's just not your style to go all out with a cat suit, opt instead for something that you'd expect to wear while prowling from bar to bar. Bold-colored shirts and tight bell-bottomed pants with your flashiest shoes will keep you looking your best no matter what back alleyway you find yourself slinking around in.

〇〇〇〇〇〇〇〇〇〇〇〇〇〇〇〇〇〇〇〇〇〇〇〇〇〇〇〇〇〇〇〇〇〇

"As a self-described professional narcissist, I think moustaches are a fascinating expression of masculinity."

— Gandhi Jones

〇〇〇〇〇〇〇〇〇〇〇〇〇〇〇〇〇〇〇〇〇〇〇〇〇〇〇〇〇〇〇〇〇〇

THE
WHIRLWIND

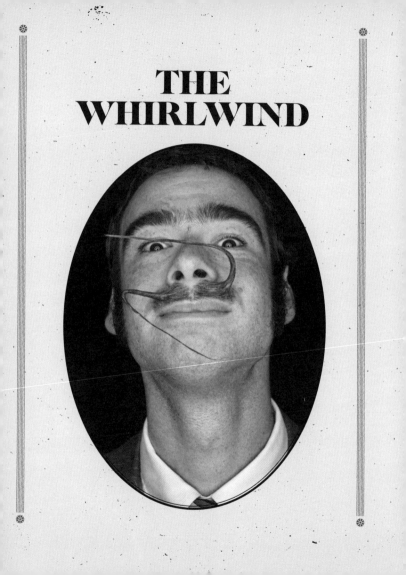

BY DEVON HOLCOMBE
MONTHS TO GROW: 6+
DIFFICULTY: 4

Aside from a striking family resemblance, Devon Holcombe shares something else with his twin brother Sam (p. 132)—a championship set of whiskers. Devon admits that his brother was the first to wear a proper moustache, but the Oklahoma-based teacher has made up for lost time by competing in various regional competitions, including placing second in the 2010 Misprint Beard and Moustache Contest in Austin, Texas. The previous year, Holcombe joined his brother at the World Beard and Moustache Championships in Anchorage. This look, which features two impressively twisted tufts of hair swooping across the face, was inspired by a style worn by Salvador Dalí and won Holcombe second place in the Freestyle Moustache category.

Begin by shaving the cheeks, neck, and chin. Allow upper-lip hair to extend approximately ½ inch past the sides of the mouth. Work a liberal amount of wax into your moustache. Wait ten to fifteen minutes for the wax to become firm yet still pliable. Use your thumb and index finger to pinch the sides of the moustache while twisting upward. Continue pinching and twisting while gradually nudging the ends into shape—one side turning directly upward and swooping horizontally just above the tip of the nose, the other side turning down and slightly out from the face before swooping in the opposite direction just below the lower lip. Use more wax if needed to keep the ends from drooping or separating.

GROOMING
Aside from regular shaving, apply wax as needed. Note: If you want to eventually transform this look into a traditional Dalí (p. 64), leave no hair extending past the sides of the mouth.

HOW TO WEAR IT
This fun, gravity-defying, and eye-catching look deserves to be dressed up, but don't overdo it with a conservative style. Choose a pinstriped suit paired with a colorful shirt and patterned tie (extra points for any pattern that complements the swoop of these whiskers). This somewhat Western look also benefits from a little frontier panache—if you have a nice pair of boots, wear them.

"If you have a moustache like this, you can't be a bad person or do bad things. People will remember you."

— Devon Holcombe

TABLE OF EQUIVALENTS

Most moustache competitions use the metric system to set guidelines for how long facial hair can be and where it can grow for any given style. Use the chart below as a quick way to convert the measurements given in this book, and be sure to check the official rules and guidelines for each competition before entering.

⅛ IN = 0.32 CM

¼ IN = 0.64 CM

½ IN = 1.27 CM

¾ IN = 1.91 CM

1 IN = 2.54 CM

2 IN = 5.08 CM

3 IN = 7.62 CM

4 IN = 10.16 CM

GROOMING

Aside from regular shaving, apply wax as needed. Note: If you want to eventually transform this look into a traditional Dalí (p. 64), leave no hair extending past the sides of the mouth.

HOW TO WEAR IT

This fun, gravity-defying, and eye-catching look deserves to be dressed up, but don't overdo it with a conservative style. Choose a pinstriped suit paired with a colorful shirt and patterned tie (extra points for any pattern that complements the swoop of these whiskers). This somewhat Western look also benefits from a little frontier panache—if you have a nice pair of boots, wear them.

"If you have a moustache like this, you can't be a bad person or do bad things. People will remember you."

— Devon Holcombe

TABLE OF EQUIVALENTS

Most moustache competitions use the metric system to set guidelines for how long facial hair can be and where it can grow for any given style. Use the chart below as a quick way to convert the measurements given in this book, and be sure to check the official rules and guidelines for each competition before entering.

⅛ IN = 0.32 CM

¼ IN = 0.64 CM

½ IN = 1.27 CM

¾ IN = 1.91 CM

1 IN = 2.54 CM

2 IN = 5.08 CM

3 IN = 7.62 CM

4 IN = 10.16 CM

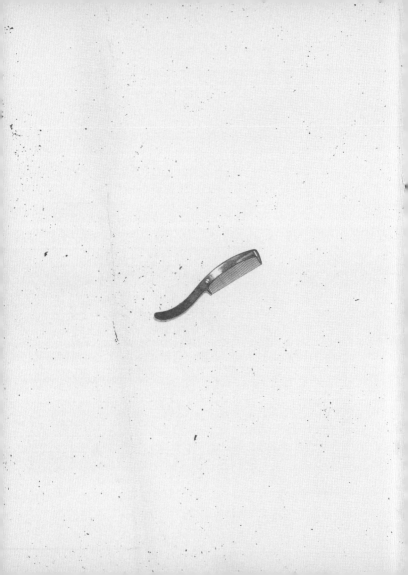